Yoga Power: Control the Energy Within

(Yoga Poses, Exercises, Stretches, Balance, Core Strength, Joint Stability, Body Awareness, Exploration, and Power)

Table of Contents

Introduction

I want to thank you and congratulate you for purchasing the book, "Yoga Power: Control the Energy Within (Yoga Poses, Exercises, Stretches, Balance, Core Strength, Joint Stability, Body Awareness, Exploration, Power)."

If you look at the way we work and live today, you will note that we spend a major portion of our time seated. Many of us hold jobs that call on us to sit at a desk and in front of a computer for more than 7 hours a day. When we get home, many of us also sit in front of the TV because watching TV has become our new way of relaxing and unwinding.

Working is great and so is relaxing. However, if you know anything about human physiology, you know that sitting causes specific muscles and joints of the body to tense up and contract, which makes movement of these muscles that much more difficult.

Additionally, when we are inactive, the muscles and tendons that stretch and shrink to allow for muscle and joint movement compact, which then causes joint and muscle atrophy.

The fact that we live in a world that seems designed for sitting does not mean we should be content with it because as research conducted by Dr. David Agus indicates that sedentary sitting for more than 5 hours is equal to smoking 1¼ packs of cigarette. The news is not all doom and gloom.

For every 20 minutes of sitting down, stand up, and for a minute or two, contract your muscles and move a little. If you sit for longer than 20 minutes at a time, you need to change that right now because after the 20-minute mark, physiological changes start to happen.

While standing up every 20 minutes is great and will help you avoid the negative effects of sitting down for too long, you should also employ other exercises that stretch and move your muscles and joints. Yoga is one such exercise—and perhaps the best form of exercise there is because in addition to helping ease out the kinks in your muscles, you can also use it as your default form of exercise in place of other exercises such as jogging, strength training and the likes.

In this guide, we shall discuss how you can make yoga a central part of your life and, by so doing, become aware of your power—and how to unleash it—stretch out your muscles, strengthen, balance and stabilize your core muscles and joints, and become aware of your body.

Yoga 101: Why Yoga–The Benefits

Being an age-old practice, yoga is more than a form of exercise for the body and joints. If practiced correctly, it also immensely benefits the mind and spirit.

Yoga has a very rich history. One aspect of this history is that Hatha yoga, the most practiced form of yoga in the modern world—we shall talk about the different types of yoga shortly—developed as a practice whose main aim was to prepare the body for the stillness of meditation.

Although the modern world treats yoga primarily as a form of exercise, it is so much more than a way to strengthen the body muscles and joints (even though these are some of its most standout benefits).

Translated, the word yoga means union: union of mind and body, a state that is achievable only when we are present in the moment as we engage in the physical aspects of hatha yoga (the yoga poses and sequences).

Why Yoga: The Benefits

Yoga has very many benefits. The most significant of these benefits are:

Improved stress control/management

Numerous scientific research studies have shown that yoga is one of the most effective ways to ease stress and anxiety. We can attribute this to the scientifically proven fact that yoga reduces the production of cortisol, the stress hormone.

One such study involved 24, emotionally distressed female participants. After engaging in a 3-month yoga program, researchers discovered a significant reduction of cortisol, a fact that led to lowered depression, stress and anxiety levels.

Yoga is most effective against stress and anxiety primarily because of its positive effect on the production of stress hormones—it decreases production of these hormones.

Improved heart health

Hatha yoga, the physical aspect of yoga and the most practiced type of yoga, will have you sweating in a short while. Because it is strenuous—in a good way of course—yoga poses will improve how effective your heart is at pumping blood to all parts of your body and thereby supplying the body with the nutrients it needs to perform optimally.

For instance, numerous studies have shown that consistent practice of yoga lowers blood pressure, which then lowers risk of heart ailments often caused by lifestyle choices such as a lack of exercise. When combined with a healthy lifestyle, yoga will have your heart (and body) operating like a well-oiled machine.

Pain Relief

A growing body of scientific research shows that yoga, perhaps thanks to its different poses/asanas, is an effective way to deal with all forms of chronic pain including pain caused by arthritis and joint injuries.

In one such study that involved 42 individuals suffering from carpal tunnel syndrome, researchers gave the participants the option of a wrist splint or yoga for 8 weeks. The study discovered that at the end of the 8 weeks period, those who practiced yoga showed decreased pain and improved grip strength. Those who went for the wrist splint showed significantly lesser results.

Better balance and flexibility

Improved balance and flexibility are one of the main reasons why many people choose to engage in yoga. To this end, considerable amounts of research prove that yoga is especially effective at optimizing balance and flexibility using very specific yoga poses.

Some research studies have shown that practicing yoga for as little as 15 minutes can improve joint and muscle performance, which will improve your balance and flexibility.

Increased strength

Because it involves physical exercise (the yoga poses/asanas are physical exercises), yoga is one of the most effective strength-building exercises there is and is a favorite because it does not involve weight lifting.

Yoga exercises such as sun salutations increase body strength and endurance and promote weight loss and lean muscle. In one such study conducted on 74 adults who performed sun salutations for 24 weeks (6 days a week), the improvements were drastic. The participants saw a massive increase in weight loss, endurance, and upper body strength. Women participating in the study also showed a massive decrease in overall body fat percentage.

These are just some of the benefits of yoga.

Now that you know the benefits of yoga and you now know why you should practice it, let us move on to discussing the different types of yoga before we move on to yoga poses and sequences.

Different Types of Yoga

Thanks to its rich history, the main yoga practiced years gone in India has branched into many different forms of yoga that we now practice. The fact that there are many types of yoga is a core hindrance to many especially those new to yoga.

Since yoga means to York or unite the mind and the body, most forms of yoga have a physical as well as mental aspect to them. While the best way to choose which type of yoga is most ideal for you is to attend a class offering beginner yoga at your local yoga studio (you will find many of these around your locality), learning a bit about the available types of yoga will help you determine which classes can accommodate you as you experiment.

Below are the common types of yoga

Hatha Yoga

Loosely translated, the term hatha yoga means all the physical aspects of yoga, i.e., the various yoga asanas you have to hold for several moments/breaths as you practice yoga. In the Western world, the term hatha is all encompassing in that it refers to all forms of yoga that have a physical element to them.

Hatha yoga is the most practiced type of yoga and is, therefore, the ideal type of yoga for beginners since it adopts slower moving sequences. Hatha yoga is also ideal because it couples forms of meditation (breathing meditation) with the yoga exercises. This is especially important because breathing meditation has many other benefits for the mind and body.

This guide is going to concentrate more on this type of yoga (the yoga poses and their sequence).

Kundalini Yoga

Kundalini yoga is part physical and spiritual. The aim of this type of yoga is the release of your Kundalini energy, a type of energy that remains coiled and trapped in your root chakra (lower spine) until you release it.

Kundalini yoga classes are fast moving; they involve core exercises (with the aim being to release the kundalini energy trapped there) and panting like breathing exercises. Some of these classes also involve an element of meditation, chakra tuning, and mantra recital/chanting.

This type of yoga is ideal for you if you are more into the spiritual aspect of yoga and want to combine it with an intense workout.

Iyengar Yoga

Founded by Bellur Krishnamachar Sundararaja Iyengar (often abbreviated as B.K.S Iyengar), this type of yoga concentrates on proper movement and alignment. In a typical Iyengar yoga class, you can expect to control your breath as you hold various yoga poses for a substantial amount of time as you align the pose in minute details.

Unlike the commonly practiced hatha yoga that often just requires a yoga mat, this type of yoga uses tons of props that aim to help you align your body to a pose. This type of yoga is very relaxing and opens all joints and muscles. It is therefore ideal for injuries and alignment.

Vinyasa Yoga

Vinyasa yoga means, "To place yoga postures in a special way." Because of its athletic nature—athletic in that it promotes flow as you move from one yoga asana to the other—this type of yoga is ideal for those looking for an intense yoga exercise while at the same time deriving the benefits of yoga.

As you move through the yoga poses, you also have to coordinate them to your breath and flow of movement from one asana to the other. Any form of yoga that promotes flow of movement and breath can also be Vinyasa yoga.

Ashtanga Yoga

Ashtanga is a Sanskrit word that loosely translates to "eight limb path." This type of yoga involves very demanding, and involving yoga poses that require an experienced hand; it, therefore, is not ideal for beginners.

With that said, this type of yoga is very rewarding in every sense of the word. Most Ashtanga yoga classes start with 5 sun salutations A's and B's before then moving to standing and floor poses performed in sequence. Like Vinyasa yoga, this type of yoga also concentrates on movement of breath and sequence.

Bikram Yoga

If your aim for practicing yoga is to sweat out all the toxicity and excess fat, this type of yoga is the perfect choice for you. Named after Bikram Choudhury, Bikram yoga happens in a sauna-like setting—or a room with a temperature of 105 degrees and 40% humidity—and includes 26 basic postures performed twice.

The above are the most basic types of yoga (and most common and popular). This does not mean these are the only types of yoga available; we have much more.

Now that you know about the different types of yoga choose one that is right for you considering your goals. What do you want to achieve with your yoga practice? While all types of yoga are beneficial, choosing one that aligns with your goals will prove most beneficial in many ways.

With that out of the way, let us discuss yoga poses that will help you achieve various goals.

Hatha Yoga Poses For Balance, Core Strength, & Joint Stability

The yoga poses we are about to illustrate are some of the most basic, and yet most effective yoga poses. These are ideal for someone just getting started in yoga. You can use these poses as the basic element of your flow yoga (Vinyasa yoga) or practice them one a time. Remember that you should hold the pose for 5-10 breaths and practice yoga every day. Are you ready to get started? Make some room and let's begin!

The Mountain Pose

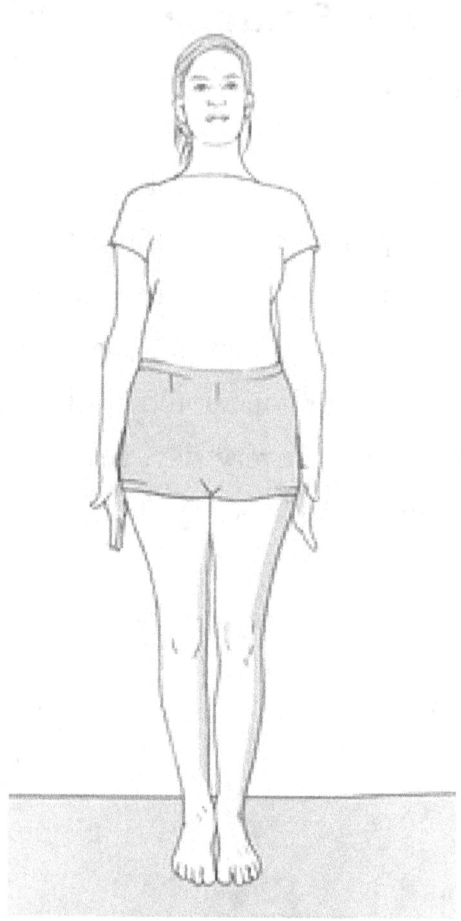

Also called Tadasana and Samasthiti, this standing yoga pose is the most basic yoga asana especially for all standing yoga asanas. This yoga pose grounds you to the earth beneath your feet.

How to get into the pose

First, there is a design to this pose—not just standing. Start with placing your feet together with your toes open and pressed into the ground. With your quadriceps engaged, lift your kneecaps up through your inner thighs. Contract your abdominals as you press your shoulders down and lift your chest up.

Open your chest widely as you contract the shoulder blades towards each other. Keep your hands by your inner thighs with the palms facing inward. Stretch the crown of your head upwards to the ceiling. Breathe deeply for 5-10 breaths.

Tree Pose

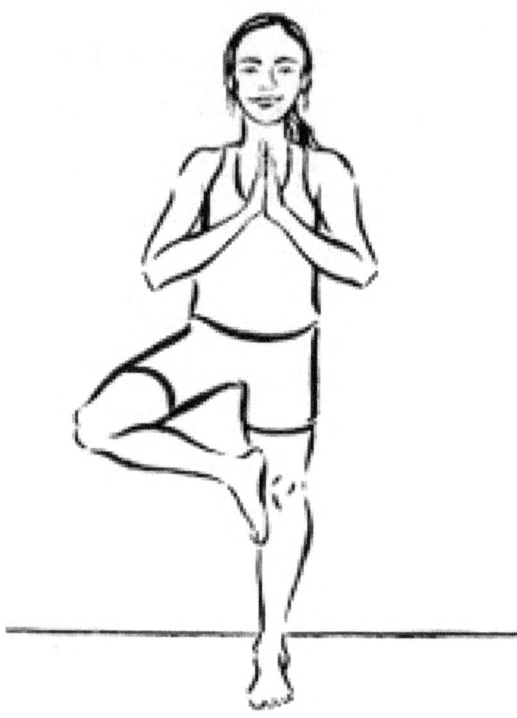

Also called Vrikshasana, this standing pose helps you develop balance, focus, and inner clarity. It also helps you focus on your breath.

How to get into the pose

From the mountain pose and with your feet placed together, lift your right foot at the knee and place the sole of the foot on the inner thigh of the other foot. Bring the palms of your hands together at the center of your chest in prayer and look ahead at a spot in front of you.

Hold that gaze to stabilize your pose. Engage your core, relax your shoulders, and keep the standing leg straight (do not lean into it). Breathe in for 8-10 breaths and then switch legs.

Triangle Pose

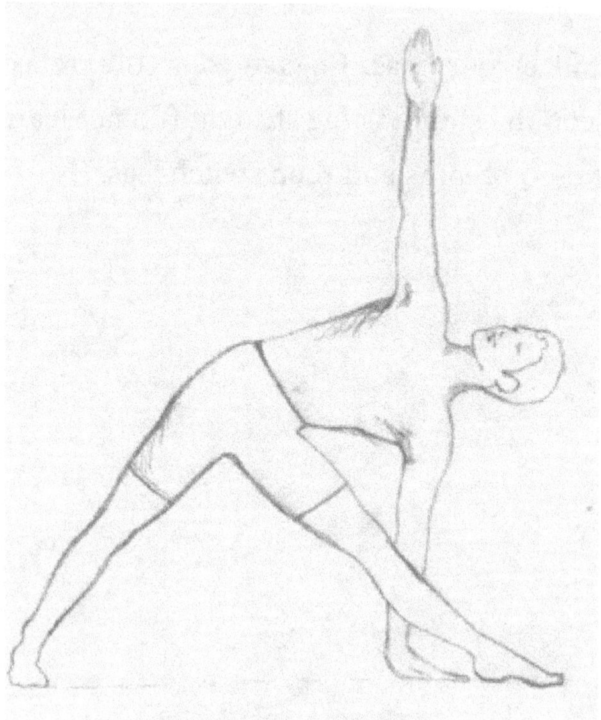

Also called Trikonasana, this standing pose tones the body stretches the waist, thighs, and shoulders, and activates and strengthens the lungs.

How to get into the pose

From the tree pose, step the leg previous on your inner thighs backward a meter or so. Stretch your hands out at shoulder height and open them. Turn your foot (preferably the right one though you are free to start with whichever side) out to a 90 degree angle with the toes of your left foot placed at a 45 degree angle.

With your abdominals and quadriceps engaged, hinge to the right and stretch your right hand to touch your knee, shin or ankle depending on your flexibility level. Lift and stretch your other hand to the ceiling and turn your gaze up to the look at the hand stretched to the ceiling.

Draw in 5-10 breathes (you can count them for a brief breath meditation session) and then lift up as you sequentially move to the other side.

Warrior 1

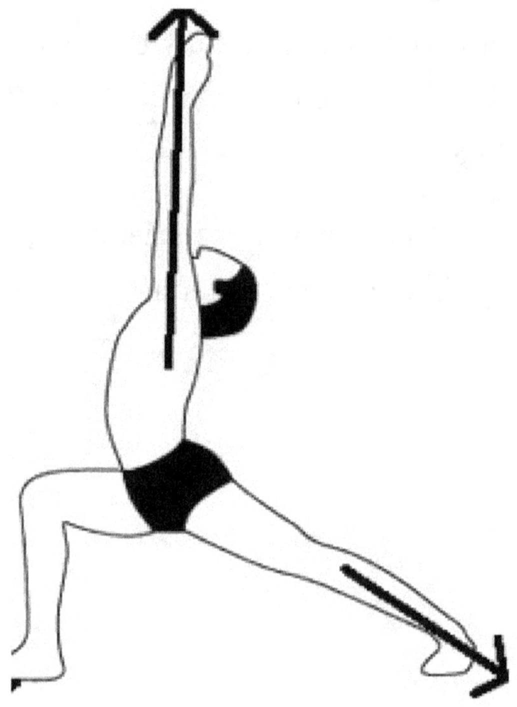

Also called Virabhadrasana I, this pose (and the one after it) builds stamina and strength. It stretches your hips and thighs; it also builds lower body and core strength. Because of the gentle bend of the back, the pose is also a very great way to stretch the lower back, the hips, buttocks, and upper body.

How to get into the pose

Assume a sort of lunge position by stepping back with your left foot. Turn the heel of your left foot down and angle the toes 75 degrees forward. Open and lift up your chest as you raise your hand above you and press them. Hold the pose for 5-10 breaths and then step forward to repeat the sequence on the other side.

Warrior 2

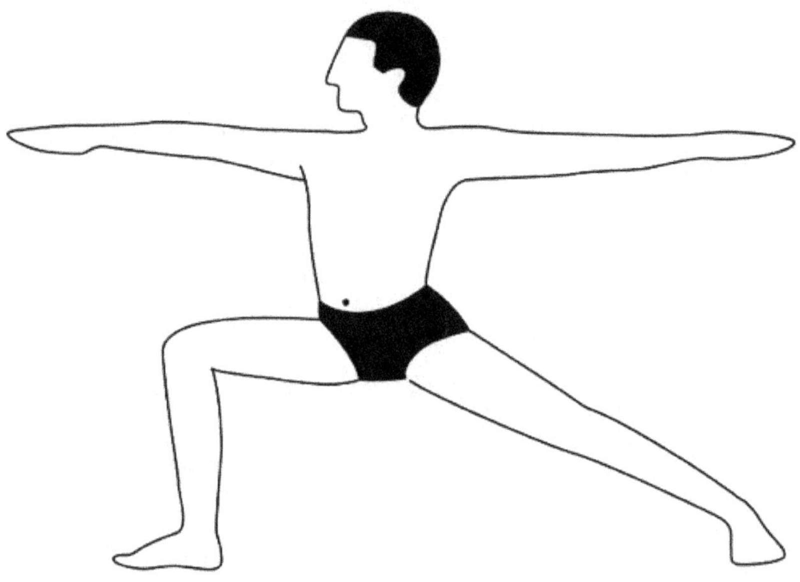

Also called Virabhadrasana II, this yoga asana stretches and opens up the hips, thighs, and groin area. Because of its positioning, this asana is especially great for transitioning into side poses such as the triangle (described below).

How to get into the pose

With your feet shoulder width apart, turn the toes of your right foot at a 90 degrees angle and those of the left foot at a 45 degrees angle. Bend the knee of the right foot until its positioning is directly over the ankle of the right foot. Keep your torso even and stabilized between the hips.

Stretch your arms as shown in the image and look ahead of the right arm. Hold the pose for 5-10 breaths depending on your level of comfort, and then straighten the right leg, turn the other foot, and then complete the sequence on the other leg.

Downward Facing Dog

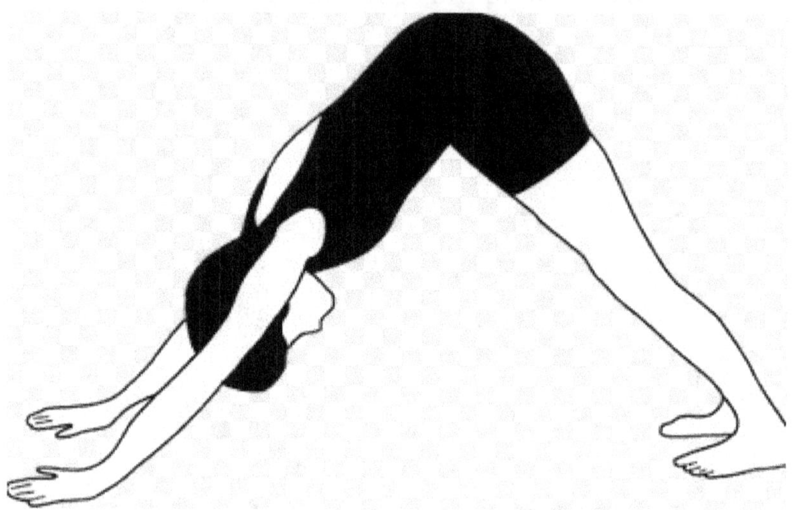

Also called Adho mukha śvānāsana, or adho mukha shvanasana, this pose is one of the most effective yoga stretches and is one of the most strengthening yoga poses.

How to get into the pose

Get on your knees and place your wrist under your knees to get into an all-fours pose; keep your knees under the hips. As you lift up at the hips, tuck in your toes and draw your hips towards the heels.

If you are not too flexible, slightly bend your knees; if you are flexible, stretch all out and keep your hips back and stable. You can also walk your hands forward to create a large triangle arch as shown in the image.

Press your palms firmly onto the ground and rotate your inner elbows until they face each other. Let your abdominals relax and to keep your torso from moving, engage your legs. Hold the pose for 5-10 breaths and then drop back on all fours.

Plank Pose

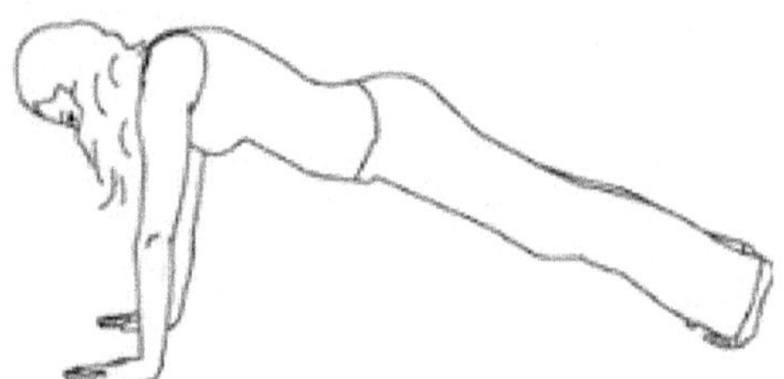

Also called Kumbhakasana (koom-bahk-AHS-uh-nuh), this yoga asana strengthens the spine, abdominals, and the arms. It is also a balancing pose aimed at fostering balance and breath control.

How to get into the pose

Get on all fours. Lift your legs off the mat making sure to keep your toes tucked. Slide back to get into a sort of push-up pose until your feet and head are in a straight line. Contract and engage your core, push your shoulders away from your ears, and breathe deeply from the diaphragm for 5-10 breaths making sure you are pulling your ribs together.

Child Pose

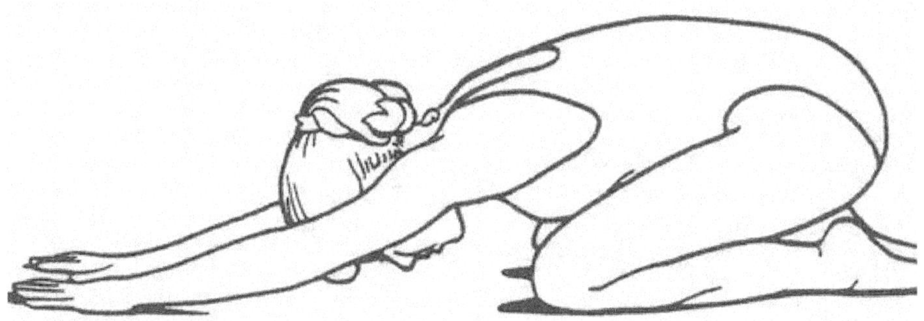

Also called Bālāsana, the child pose is one of the most relaxing yoga poses. This pose will offer you immense relaxation and stress relief especially if you practice it before bed as a way to unwind after a long day. The pose is so easy that anyone can practice it.

How to get into the pose

Get on all fours. Pull your knees close together, sit back on your heels, and stretch your arms before you. Touch the yoga mat with your forehead and then let your body loose. Hold the pose for 8-10 breaths or for as long as you want.

Seated Forward Bend

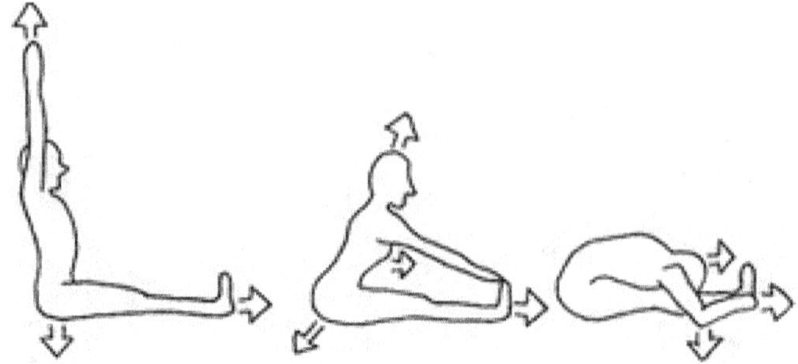

Also called Paschimottanasana or Intense Dorsal Stretch, this pose stretches out your sides, hamstrings, and entire back. Because of the intricate bend of the pose, it teaches you how to breathe properly as you work through difficult yoga positions.

As a contraindication of adopting this pose, be mindful of any painful experiences. If you note a sharp pain, ease off. However, if you can breathe despite the tension of the bend, continue holding the fold for as long as you want—8-10 breaths will do—so that your body can start loosening.

How to get into the pose

Start from a sitting position with your legs placed together, hands beside your hips, and your feet flexed with the heels on the mat and toes pointed upwards and to the ceiling and stretched. If you are not too flexible, you can bend your knees as long as you make sure the feet are together and flexed.

As you start to bend forward at the waist, open your chest and engage your abdominal muscles. Once you can bend no more, hold the pose for 5-10 breaths making sure to relax your head, shoulders, and chest.

Bridge Pose

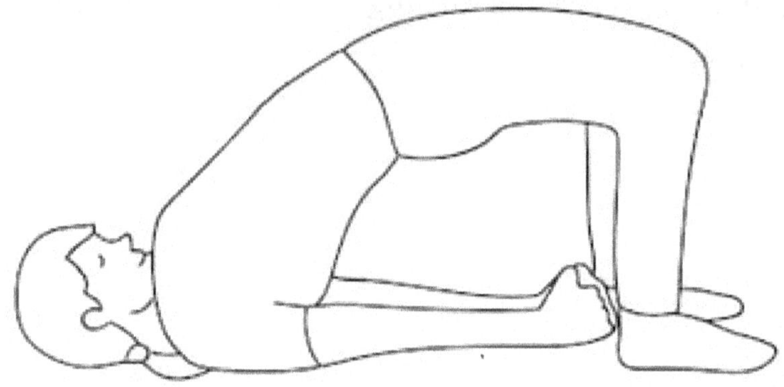

Also called Setu Bandha Sarvangasana, this yoga asana is a backbend that strengthens and stretches the back and front body. Specifically, this pose stretches and opens up the spine and aligns the upper and middle back.

How to get into the pose

Start in a lying down position with your back placed firmly on your yoga mat with your feet placed hip width apart. Press the soles of your feet into the ground as you hinge upward at the waist and lift your butt up into the air. Bring your hands together under your butt and interlace them with the fists pressed into the floor as you open up your chest. Engage your hamstrings and hold the pose for 8-10 deep breaths. Lower down to the floor and repeat the sequence 3-5 times.

With these 10 yoga poses, you can start your yoga journey with ease. Obviously, because we have tones of yoga asanas, it is impossible to list all yoga asanas here. Once you start doing these basic yoga poses, you can move to other more advanced poses.

Vinyasa Yoga For Body Awareness, Exploration, & Power

Vinyasa yoga or flow yoga is a sequential type of yoga that unlike Hatha yoga that concentrates on individual poses, concentrates on the smooth flow of poses stringed together to form a sequence.

Sun salutations are one of the key elements of flow yoga. You can use the poses of Vinyasa as a form of warm up or as part of your full yoga practice. Learning a Vinyasa yoga sequence will complement what you have learned that far and because this type of yoga concentrates on flow, you will become intimately aware of your body and how it moves from one asana to the other.

Vinyasa yoga pays very special attention to the flow of breath and as you will coordinate your breath with movement from one pose to the next, i.e., you will coordinate your inhalation and exhalations with movement from asana to asana, which means moving to the next asana with the correct breath.

The following Vinyasa yoga sequence will prove very helpful as a warm up or for body awareness, exploration, or power.

If you are enjoying this book, would you be kind enough to leave a review on Amazon because I would like to hear how the book has improved your life. If you make it to the last page of this book and did not enjoy its value, publisher details will be given to inform what could have been done to better serve your expectations.

Step 1: Mountain Pose

Start in the mountain pose (you already know how to execute the mountain pose).

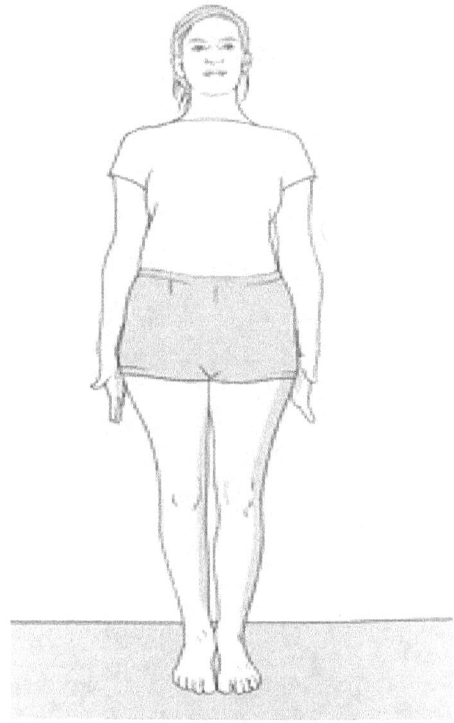

The mountain pose is normally the traditional starting and stopping point of sun salutations. Raise your hands up from the sides of your body to the ceiling and join the palms. Lift your eyes to watch your thumbs and push your shoulders down and away from your ears.

Step 2: Mountain Pose To Flat Back

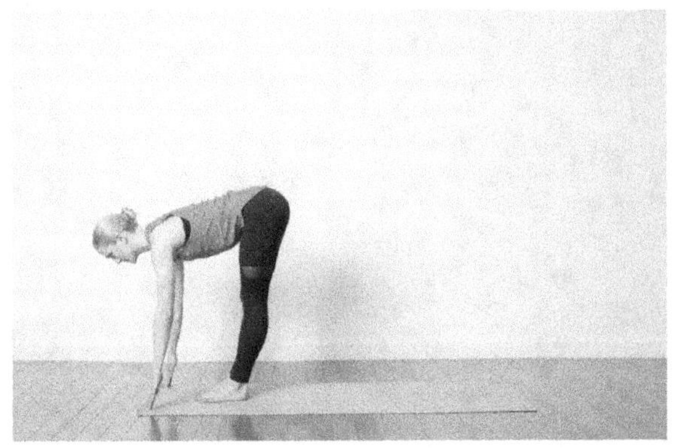

As you exhale, hinge forward at the waist with your legs straight as if you are about to dive into a swimming pool.

Inhale and touch the floor with the toes in line with the fingers, and if you are flexible enough, press your palms into the floor. If you are not that flexible and your palms do not reach the floor, use blocks. Raise your head to get into the flat back and keep your back aligned and straight.

Step 3: Flat Back To Plank

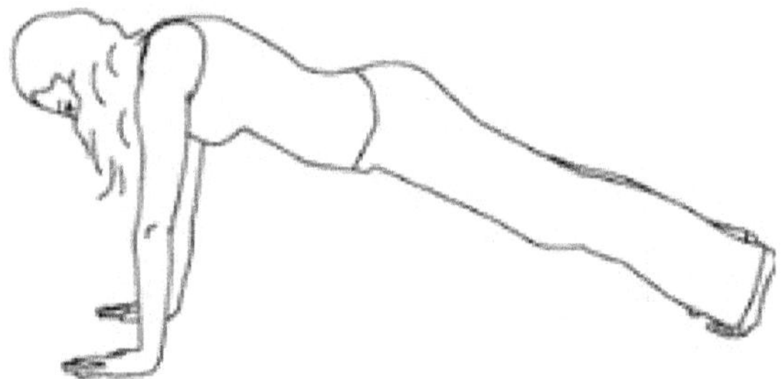

From the flat back, exhale as you press your palms into the mat and jump back to get into the plank pose. After jumping back, align your shoulder to be over your wrists, tighten your abs, and keep the butt straight and in line with the rest of the body. Imagine a straight line between the top of your head and your heels. Once aligned, take a deep breath.

Step 4: Plank To Four-Limbed Staff Pose

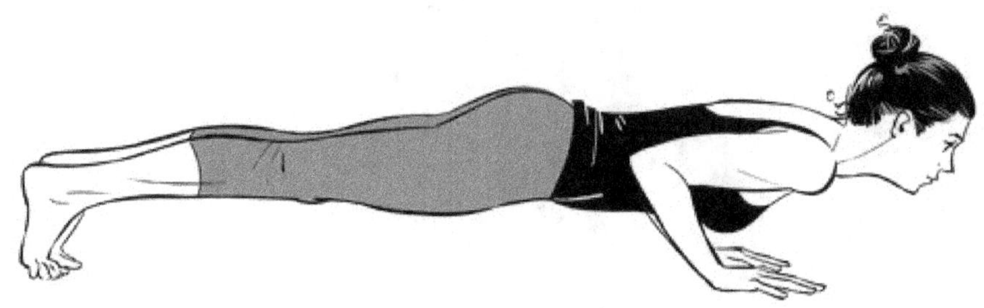

While in the plank pose, exhale and lower your knees and chest. Lower the chest to the floor in a sort of pushup stance, and align your shoulders over your hands. Lift your butt high and press your elbows into your ribs with the elbows in line with the shoulders and heels.

If you are a bit more flexible and advanced in your yoga journey, from the plank pose, exhale and move your shoulders forward in front of your wrists before you lower yourself into the four-limbed staff pose and align yourself in the final pose. Be mindful of shoulder injuries (make sure you are doing the pose correctly).

Step 5: Four-Limbed Staff Pose To Cobra Pose

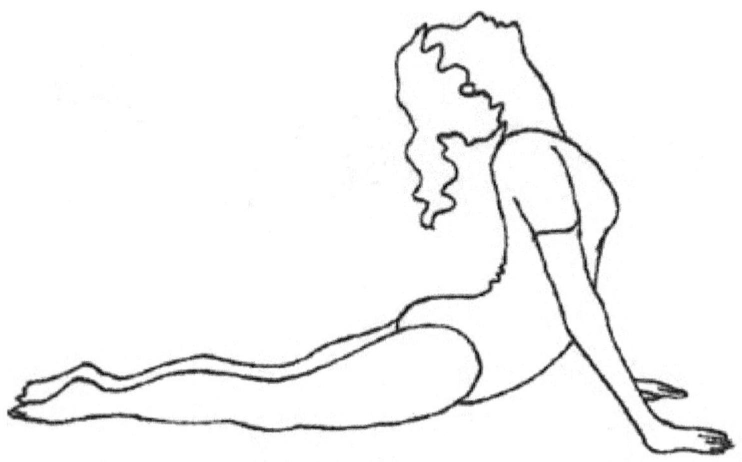

While in the four-limbed pose, inhale deeply and then lower your waist to the floor to get into the low cobra pose. Press the tops of your feet and your pelvis to the floor and with your palms pressed into the floor (not too hard though), come into a backbend.

If you were in the more advanced pose described in the previous step, inhale deeply, and bend your elbows to make sure your shoulders and ears are away from each other. Once in this pose, straighten your arms making sure your legs and knees are straight and off the floor.

Step 6: Cobra Pose To Downward Facing Dog

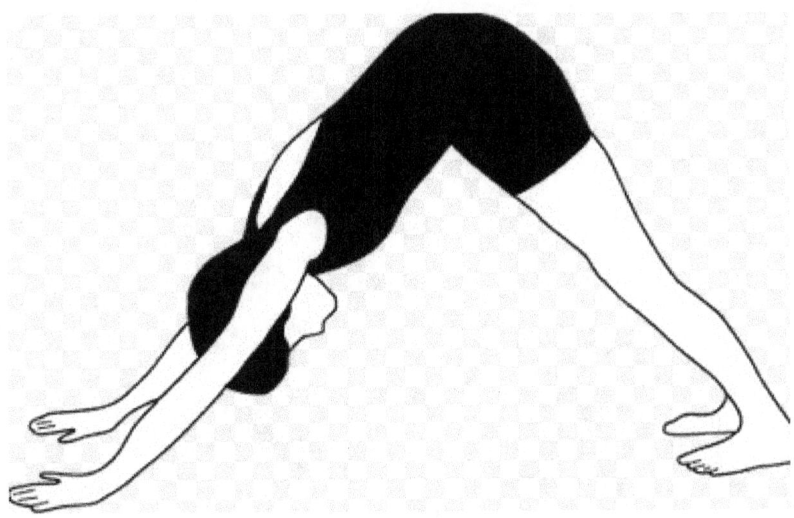

While in the cobra pose, exhale deeply and push through your hands to come into the downward facing dog pose. Hold this pose for several minutes or breaths or one breath depending on your pace.

Step 7: Downward Dog To Standing Forward Bend

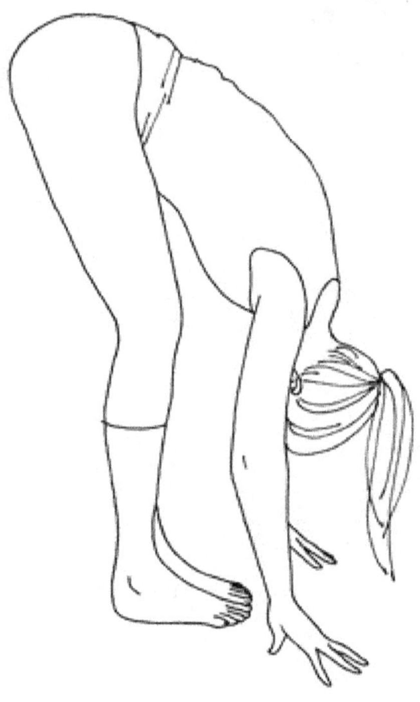

While in the downward dog, exhale deeply and step or jump into the forward bend. You can do this by stepping either one of your foot to the corresponding hand and then bringing the other to join to get into the forward bend as described earlier. If you opt to jump forward, exhale as you bend your knees and jump to bring the feet and hands together making sure to land with your toes and fingertips aligned.

Inhale into the flat back and then exhale into the Intense Forward-Bending Pose by pushing your head into your shins and holding onto the back of your legs

Step 8: Mountain Pose

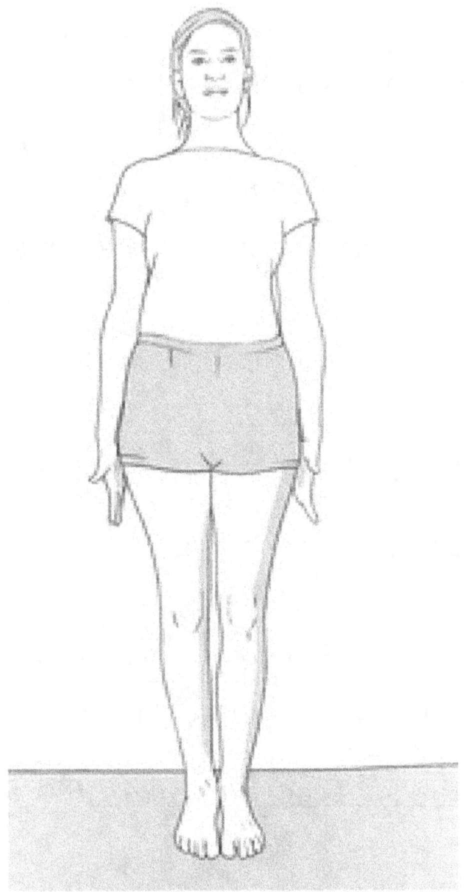

Exhale deeply as you come into the mountain pose with your hands at your sides.

Advanced: Ashtanga Yoga Poses

After Hatha Yoga, Ashtanga Yoga is one of the classical kinds of yoga. It's considered by many solid yoga practitioners to be a meticulous and serious form of yoga. Ashtanga Yoga's form is made up of yoga poses that involve relatively challenging positions like inversions, twists, and backbends. The Asanas of Ashtanga Yoga involve flowing movements and rhythmic breaths that help heat up the body's deep core. They also help in cleansing the soul, mind, and body. We'll take a look at the basic Ashtanga Yoga poses first before diving into the more advanced ones.

Basic Ashtanga Yoga Postures

Baddha Konasana: The Bound Angle Posture

1. Begin by sitting tall and upright on your mat.
2. Exhale, fold in your knees and let your heels touch each other before pulling them in the direction of your pelvis. To secure your feet, clasp your hands around them.

Prasarita Padottanasana: The Wide-Legged Forward Bend Posture

1. Begin by standing on your mat, feet about 3-inches away from each other, with your hands on your butt.
2. Maintaining a torso that's higher than your back, exhale (keep the torso length) and lean your torso forward at

the hips. Let your arms hang down with your wrists directly beneath your shoulders.

3. If you can, let the top of your head rest on the floor without letting go of your breath.

<u>Sarvangasana: The Shoulder Stand Posture</u>

1. Begin by lying straight on your mat. Your arms must be positioned at the sides.

2. Bring your heels close to the hip area by bending at the knees.

3. Press the palm of your hands on the mat for support and raise bring your thighs close to your chest by raising your feet and legs.

4. Continue raising both feet and legs to bring your knees closer to your head, supporting your weight and keeping a steady posture using your hands pressed on the mat.

5. Gradually extend your knees (straighten) and let your thighs become perpendicular to your torso, with your heels completely lifted up towards the ceiling.

<u>Utthita Hasta Padangustasana: The Hand-to-Big-Toe Posture</u>

1. Begin by assuming the basic mountain pose with your hands resting on your hips.

2. Bring your left leg to your stomach and hold the outer side of your left foot tightly.

3. Inhale while stretching your left leg as forward as you possibly can. Stability will come from the tension between your arm and foot.

4. If you want a deeper posture or stronger pull, turn your head to your left side.

5. Do the same for the other (right) side.

Utkatasana: The Chair Posture

1. Begin by standing upright with both feet close together.

2. Breathe in and stretch your arms above you in a parallel position with palms facing each other inward.

3. Exhale and bend your knees. Lean your torso slightly forward over your thighs.

4. Keep your shoulder blades steady and lower back straight throughout the posture.

Advanced Ashtanga Yoga Postures

Urdhva Kukkutasana: The Upward Rooster Posture

1. Begin by assuming the dolphin pose.

2. Bring your feet in by walking them in. Position your knees on your upper arms then hug yourself into a small package.

3. Bring your hips and tightly draw your thighs towards your chest. To help you achieve a good center of gravity, keep yourself as compact as possible.

4. After every couple of breaths, be cognizant to keep your elbows in and your shoulders lifted.

5. As soon as your hips are stacked over your shoulders, you'll feel the weight of your legs becoming substantially lighter and that your core will be able to connect.

6. Pull your knees off the arms lightly by hooking through the lower abdomen so you can assume a pike position in your chest.

7. Always maintain contact between your big toes and inner heels as you raise your legs up to the ceiling, like being sucked inside a straw.

8. Embrace your inner thighs up to the midline, widen through your kneecaps' backs, and spread out your toes.

9. Transition into the Upside-Down Lotus Posture (Sirasana).

10. Before proceeding from this posture, ensure that your foundation is strong and stable. Ensure that your shoulders are lifted to ease pressure on the neck and that your elbows should be in over your wrists.

11. Begin to fold your lotus into your body until both knees are resting on your arms. As soon as your knees land

on your arms, begin "walking" them up your arms like a small ladder.

12. Wiggle one leg to your underarm first, followed by the other leg. Make sure that you've snuggled both legs into your armpits as deep as you possibly can.

13. Reestablish connection with your shoulders' lift while keeping your core nice and tight.

14. Begin to press your knees' weight onto your arms while you bring the hips back to the ground. At this point, you'll be in a deep fold, which can make you feel so heavy. At this point, take your time.

15. When you're ready, push deeply into your palms, with your fingers lightly digging in to assist in pulling your chest forward.

16. As soon as you feel your weight shift in your hips, begin to roll from the top of your head towards your hairline. Push the ground away as soon as your eyes meet the ground or the mat.

17. As you continue elevating your posture, keep your eyes looking forward. Your arms will become straighter as you push the ground due to the round in your back.

18. Keep your torso and Lotus as tight as possible while taking 5 breaths.

19. To release, you can either bend your elbows so you can return to a headstand or slide down your arms like a fireman sliding down a firepole for fun.

<u>*Vishvamitrasana*</u>

1. Begin by inhaling and bringing your arms above your head.
2. Exhale, spread your fingers and then bend your upper body forward hinged at your hips until your hands touch the ground. Keep your lower back straight at all times.
3. Inhale as you extend your torso halfway back up or until parallel to the ground. Raise your head.
4. Place your hands on the floor, float your feet backward to form a plank, and position your elbows near your chest to assume the Chaturanga Dandasana Posture.
5. Inhale, support your body weight using the tops of your feet, straighten your arms, and extend your body as far back as possible to assume the Urdhva Mukha Shvanasana posture.
6. Exhale, push the balls of your feet against the floor, push your hands and arms against the floor, lift your hips back and up, and straighten your arms to assume the Adho Mukha Shvanasana.
7. Inhale and place your right leg over your right arm. Exhale and place your left arm on your side, using your right hand to balance your body. Inhale then extend your right leg and raise your left arm to assume the Vishvamitrasana Posture.

8. Exhale, return your left hand to rest on your side, then to the ground.

9. Inhale and lift both of your legs.

10. Exhale, gradually lower yourself and keep your elbows close to your body to return to the Chaturanga Dandasana posture.

11. Inhale, support your lower body weight with the tops of your feet, open up your torso, and extend your arms to assume the Urdhva Mukha Shvanasana posture.

12. Tuck in your toes, push your hands against the ground, bring your hips back and up with arms fully extended to assume the Adho Mukha Shvanasana posture as you exhale.

13. Bring your left leg over your left arm as you inhale.

14. Exhale, let your right arm lie on your side and balancing your body using your left hand.

15. Inhale, extend your left leg, and raise up your right arm.

16. Exhale, bring yourself down slowly while keeping your elbows close to your side to assume the Chaturanga Dandasana posture.

17. Inhale and assume the Urdhva Mukha Shvanasana posture again by shifting your lower body weight to the tops of your fee, opening up your torso, and extending your arms fully.

18. Exhale and assume the Adho Mukha Shvanasana posture once again by tucking your toes in, pushing

back against the ground with your hands, bringing your hips back and up, and keeping your hands fully extended.

19. Inhale and in one sudden motion, jump your feet in between your hands (still pressed against the floor), straightening your back halfway up, and raising your head.

20. Exhale, draw in your chest completely to assume the Uttanasana posture.

21. Inhale, raise your head yet again and straighten your back, with your palms still pressing against the ground.

22. Exhale and bring yourself up to a straight standing position with arms to the side to assume the Samasthitih posture and conclude the session.

Cakorāsana

1. Begin by lifting your arms above your head. Inhale as you do.

2. Spread your fingers then bend your torso forward from the waistline, keeping your lower back and legs straight all throughout until your hands touch the ground to assume the Uttanasana posture. Exhale as you do.

3. Inhale, raise your torso halfway back up or until parallel to the ground, keeping your lower back straight all throughout, and lift your head.

4. Put your hands down on the ground (pressing against the floor), bring your feet as far back as possible with your elbows as close to your chest as possible to assume the Chaturanga Dandasana posture. Exhale as you do.

5. Inhale, support your lower body's weight with the tops of your feet, open up your chest, extend your arms fully, and bend backward as far as you can to assume the Urdvha Mukha Shvanasana posture.

6. Exhale and assume the Adho Mukha Shvanasana posture once again by tucking your toes in, pushing back against the ground with your hands, bringing your hips back and up, and keeping your hands fully extended.

7. Inhale, then leap forward. Balance your entire body using your fully extended arms with your legs raised from the floor in a bent manner. Exhale, and swing your right leg over your right arm and behind your head as you descend to the ground.

8. Inhale, bring your body up to assume the Chakorasana posture. Take 5 breaths while maintaining the posture. Inhale while swinging your body up and back.

9. Bring your body down gradually with your elbows touching the side of your body to assume the Chaturanga Dandasana posture. Exhale as you do.

10. Inhale, support your lower body's weight with the tops of your feet, open up your chest, extend your arms fully,

and bend backward as far as you can to assume the Urdvha Mukha Shvanasana posture.

11. Exhale and assume the Adho Mukha Shvanasana posture once again by tucking your toes in, pushing back against the ground with your hands, bringing your hips back and up, and keeping your hands fully extended.

12. Inhale, then leap forward. Balance your entire body using your fully extended arms with your legs raised from the floor in a bent manner. Exhale, and swing your left leg over your left arm and behind your head as you descend to the ground.

13. Inhale, bring your body up to assume the Chakorasana posture. Take 5 breaths while maintaining the posture. Inhale while swinging your body up and back.

14. Bring your body down gradually with your elbows touching the side of your body to assume the Chaturanga Dandasana posture. Exhale as you do.

15. Inhale, support your lower body's weight with the tops of your feet, open up your chest, extend your arms fully, and bend backward as far as you can to assume the Urdvha Mukha Shvanasana posture.

16. Exhale and assume the Adho Mukha Shvanasana posture once again by tucking your toes in, pushing back against the ground with your hands, bringing your

hips back and up, and keeping your hands fully
extended.

17. Inhale and with hands planted on the ground, make
your feet leap between your hands, straighten your back
halfway, and raise your head.

18. Exhale, draw your chest in completely while inhaling to
assume the Uttanasana posture. Inhale, raise your head
yet again, and fully straighten or extend your back while
your palms remain planted on the floor. Exhale, then
stand up completely with your arms by your side to
assume the Smasthitih posture to conclude.

Pranayama Breathing: Yoga To Control The Energy & Power Within

As you may have noted, yoga is part exercise and part meditation because on top of the stretches and poses, it also asks you to become aware of your breath as you move through the poses.

Pranayama breathing while engaging in yoga is one of the most effective ways to restore your worn out energy. It renews and sustains your energy and power. Pranayama breathing simply entails breath control, which we shall now illustrate how to do as you practice yoga.

Pranayama breathing (or breath control) is the fourth of the eight limbs of yoga.

Prana (as in Pranayama) means the vital life force that sustains all living things. By practicing proper breathing exercises that target the control of breath, you can cleanse the body and mind and therefore increase your energy and improve your health and wellbeing.

Traditional yoga offers different breathing techniques; modern day yoga classes, however, concentrate more on the following yogic breath technique with the guidance of a yoga teacher.

Dirga Pranayama or Three-part Breath

This is the most basic yogic breath technique taught to all beginner yogis. It fosters awareness of the present moment and calms the mind and body. Since it does not require special preparations, you can practice it at any time.

How to practice three-part breath

Get into a comfortable yoga asana such as the corpse pose (lie on your back) or the easy pose. Place one hand on your belly and the other on your rib cage. Close your eyes and breathe naturally. Focus on your breath; watch how it moves to and from your body. Feel the hand on your belly lift up and how the rib cage expands to accommodate the expansion of the lungs as you breathe in; feel how they compress inwards as you exhale.

Move the hand on your belly to the area just below your collarbone. Take a deep breath into this area and notice how your chest rises even so slightly. Exhale and as you do, note the minute changes in this area of the body.

Watch again as your belly lifts and the ribs expand on the in-breath as well as how the chest lifts. As you exhale, note the drop in your chest, belly, and how your rib cage contracts. Let your hands drop to your side and focus fully on the experience of breathing.

Ujjayi Pranayama or Ocean Breath

This pose also calms the mind and is therefore very beneficial to energy control since it helps ease mental tension and insomnia. You will notice it practiced frequently in Vinyasa and Ashtanga yoga classes because it helps practitioner stay calm, present, and warm throughout the practice.

How to practice three-part breath

Get into a comfortable yoga pose such as the easy pose. Once settled and comfortable, inhale deeply through the mouth and be one with the experience of the air as it passes through your windpipe and down to its final resting place.

To exhale, contract the back of your throat, as you would when whispering; visualize your breath being a fog. Keep the throat contracted as you exhale and inhale deeply for 5-10 breaths and thereafter start breathing through your nose. Focus on the sound made by the breath as it travels in and outside you; it will have a very calming effect on you.

Observer as your breath fills your lungs and expands the rib cage and chest, as well as the effect on the exhalation on the body. Make the movement of your in and out-breath one with the movement of your body.

Yogic breath exercises are potent ways to align the mind and the body as you practice your yoga poses (especially when you are in the calming yoga poses such as child and easy pose).

Conclusion

Thank you again for purchasing this book.

As you have learned, yoga is very beneficial provided you do it consistently and in the right way. Before you start practicing, consult your doctor and seek the guidance of a qualified yogi at least for your first several classes.

Please remember to leave your review on Amazon if you enjoyed this book.

Thank you and good luck!